Diary Of An Imprisoned Mind

Jennifer Orsak and Amy Hurley

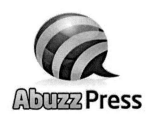

Abuzz Press

Copyright © 2016 Jennifer Orsak and Amy Hurley

ISBN: 978-1-63263-955-4

Library of Congress Cataloguing in Publication Data
Orsak, Jennifer
Diary of an Imprisoned Mind by Jennifer Orsak
Fiction / Medical | Medical / Geriatrics | Family & Relationships /
    Life Stages / Later Years
Library of Congress Control Number: 2016908458

Published by BookLocker.com, Inc., Bradenton, Florida.

Printed on acid-free paper.

The characters and events in this book are fictitious. Any similarity to real persons, living or dead, is coincidental and not intended by the author.

BookLocker.com, Inc.
2016

First Edition

Introduction

One afternoon approximately twenty years ago, a gentleman stopped and asked to speak to someone in charge of the skilled nursing facility where I worked as the assistant director of nursing.

Walking up to him, I introduced myself and asked, "How can I help you?"

"I just thought you might want to know there is an elderly person walking on the side of the road about a half mile from here. They are partially dressed in pajamas and I worried it might be someone who lives here."

The gentleman truly appeared to be concerned. My heart picked up about forty beats and my stomach turned to knots. Our facility was equipped with a system which should have alarmed if one of the wandering residents had exited the building. Having worked with the elderly for a long time though, I knew there was always a risk that something might happen and a resident could leave.

My mind went through different scenarios. "Was it indeed our resident? Had the alarm bracelet failed? Had our door failed to alarm? Had a staff member ignored the alarm and reset it without searching appropriately to assure no one exited? Had we not appropriately identified someone as a wanderer and subsequently the person just walked away quietly?"

I quickly gave notice for all units to make rounds immediately and verify all residents were present. Then I obtained the assistance of one of my employees and drove my car to the location where the concerned gentleman had last reported seeing the elderly person walking.

Within a few moments I spied an elderly man walking on the side of the road. I pulled over to better identify if indeed the gentleman was one of our residents. I did not recognize the person. Our rather large facility was home to 149 residents. I was familiar with all the long term residents but our rehabilitation unit often had multiple admissions and discharges on a daily basis. Although I tried to stay abreast of the new admissions I wanted to assure this was not one of our new residents whom I had not yet met. I looked to my fellow employee and felt my panic beginning to subside slightly as she shook her head back and forth. Thankfully she was signifying that the person was not one of our newer residents either. I was still concerned though and got out of the car to speak to the elderly man.

"Are you okay?" I asked after introducing myself.

The elderly person was attired partially in pajamas as the concerned gentleman had noted earlier. Fortunately the weather was not extreme. After conversing with the elderly person for a while I found that he resided in close proximity and had nearly completed his walk to his home. Although apparently quite eccentric he didn't appear confused or at risk of danger.

I wished him well and returned to the facility, but I will always remember the panic that arose when I thought we might have failed in assuring the safety of one of our vulnerable residents.

Throughout my career I mainly worked with geriatric patients. The majority of patients and residents whom I encountered suffered from some degree of memory loss. In my years of work I saw individuals with varied degrees of confusion and behaviors. One thing became clear in those years. Dementia does not discriminate. It strips the dignity of all afflicted regardless of a person's socioeconomic status, race, or education. The saintly neighbor around the corner who is known to be the community charitable workhorse may one day curse, hit, and spit at almost anyone they encounter. They might sit quietly hour after hour wasting away while refusing to eat and mumbling what appears to be unintelligible words and odd phrases. They might steal, hoard, pace, and wander. They may refuse to shower and change clothes. They may be able to hide their confusion quite well and appropriately converse for a lengthy time before suddenly making a remark which alerts you that they are not oriented after all. They may beg to go home and try time after time after time to get there.

So what is going through their minds as they display such extremes of passive and aggressive behavior? What do they really intend to say when they only mumble an intelligible sound? Why do they hit a total stranger without any provocation? Why do tears suddenly flood their eyes? Why do they refuse a caregiver's help? Why do they ask you the same question over and over and over again?

Unfortunately in recent years my own mother was diagnosed with a form of dementia. I talked to her almost daily. At times I felt her inner struggle as she was trying to make sense of her world. When she was initially diagnosed one of the hardest things was to observe how adamant she was in her conviction she was fine and needed no help. As many individuals she had become quite skilled in hiding her developing confusion. As time progressed and she also experienced delusions, it became even sadder. With the same degree of certainty that most of us can look up and declare the sky to be blue, my mother was equally convinced her ideations were real. Her thoughts provided her with the evidence.

Some people estimate on average a normal human being will experience 70,000 thoughts per day. Although individuals who are afflicted with dementia are confused, their mind is still working through thousands of thoughts every day just like our mind. Whereas our thoughts allow us to generally function and enjoy life, their thoughts form a chaotic and constant struggle which is unfathomable to us.

What if they could convey their inner struggle? What would they say to us? Would there be more sympathy and an increased effort to cure Alzheimer's disease and other related dementia disorders if we were able to read their confused minds?

As caregivers we often feel a surge of adrenaline and concern when we sense that a confused individual is in serious immediate danger. As in the initial scenario regarding the pajama clad elderly man, I felt the heightened awareness to act because I recognized that horrific things could happen. If the gentleman had been a wandering resident and subsequently killed by a passing car then his death would have been viewed as a tragic incident.

It is my hope this fictional story will create this same heightened awareness in people regarding the tragedy these confused individuals experience on a daily basis as they battle the conflicts and thoughts in their minds. Their day to day struggle could be considered horrific. Hopefully the story will also increase respect for caregivers and the immense challenges they face while caring for individuals who suffer from dementia.

The story is written hypothetically based on years of dealing with confused individuals who exhibited an array of behaviors. It centers on a fictional character, Irene. Before you read it I ask you to think about the most cherished individual in your life; your mother, father, husband, wife, child, or friend. Then I ask you to consider, "What if this story was the real diary of your loved one?"

Would your heart rate increase forty beats? Would you have the adrenaline rush to get started and try to make a difference? Would you become more involved in contributing to Alzheimer's and dementia research and awareness? Would you take a little more time when you next encounter someone who is confused and anxious?

In the following pages may you feel Irene's struggle and pain as you live within her mind during a period of one day in a facility where she has resided for several years. May you experience her frustration as she grasps to make sense of her world and feels fully justified when she hits, wanders, curses, refuses care, silently accuses others of untrue things, and attempts to go home. May you find that her muttered unintelligible phrases hold true meaning in her confused mind. As you live her struggle may you develop empathy for an incurable process which steals the dignity of over five million individuals and for whom the afflicted have difficulty speaking for themselves. May you hear their weary cries knowing they live similar circumstances of the following day over and over and over again.

Irene's story

Looking out the window I silently tell myself, "I must hurry. I must hurry. I must hurry!!"

The sun is beginning to rise now, and I see what my eyes have been searching to find. I spy my car parked three spaces from my window view. I see no one else in the parking lot. It is the opportune time. I must hurry.

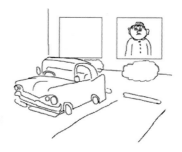

Walking quickly back to the bed I bend over my open suitcase and haphazardly throw more items into it. Did I get everything? I slowly straighten up. My back catches in a sharp pain as it tries to cooperate. I try to ignore the pain and be optimistic. Today will be a good day. Today I am going home and no one will stop me.

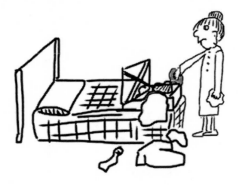

The catch in my back is becoming a little more intense. Oh, my arthritis. Of all days, why did it pick this one to act up? I'll just take one moment and go to my bathroom medicine cabinet to retrieve my Tylenol. That should fix it.

Walking away from my suitcase I enter the bathroom, pick up a cup, and prepare to fill it with water. I turn on the faucet and look around. My medicine cabinet is gone. But where is it? It has always been here. Something isn't right. I drop my water cup on the floor and ignore the water which continues to run. I look around in a panic. What have they done with my medicine?

I instinctively grab my head. "Think Irene. Think." I silently coax myself.

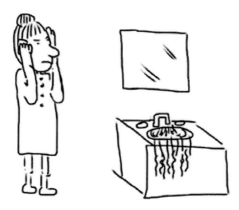

For a moment I thought this was my bathroom, but it isn't. My medicine is at home. Home!! That is it. My mind rushes. I must get home. Paying no heed to the water that continues to run in the bathroom sink I leave the bathroom and approach the bed once again.

"She will be here. She will be here," I repeat silently to myself.

My daughter left me here a few days ago. How could she have done this to me? That conniving stealing little wench-who would have thought? After all those years of raising and taking care of her and now to find all she wants is my money-my house and my bank account. I am fine and I will prove it. I will be gone from this horrible place when she comes back to check on me. But I must hurry. She will be here. I would have never, never, never thought in a million years she would do this….never…never….never...

Once again I instinctively grab my head to stop my thoughts.

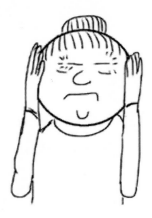

If I could just get home to a quiet place I will be able to think clearly. I am sure of it. There. I will just give my suitcase a final snap and everything is quite tidy and ready to go.

From habit I glance in the mirror before leaving. It appears I may need just a tad of lipstick. Now where did I place that? Did I pack it? Opening my suitcase once again, I rummage through hastily. Hum…It's not here. Maybe I left it in a drawer. I walk to the dresser again and pull open a drawer to search.

Oh my, what is all this?

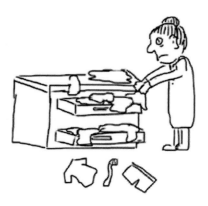

I must have missed quite a few things when packing. I thought for sure I put everything in my suitcase. I ruffle through. These things certainly do not belong to me. I never wear such things. Wonder where they came from? Well, I will deal with that later. I must find that lipstick!! To no avail, I am not able to locate my missing cosmetic. Leaving the drawer half open I apprehensively walk back to the window to make sure my car is still there. What if my daughter came and got my car while I was searching for that stupid lipstick?

Becoming apprehensive I murmur aloud as I gaze out the window, "Spoodles and tunes. Spoodles and tunes. Spoodles and tunes."

Yes, there it is. My car is still there. I can't wait to go home.

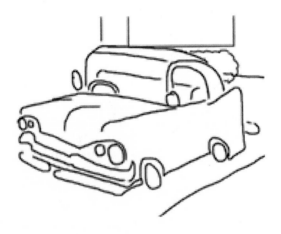

Spoodles and tunes. Oh, I'll just forget that stupid lipstick. I return to the bed once again and slam my luggage shut. I give it a huge heave and prepare to lift when suddenly there is a knock at the door.

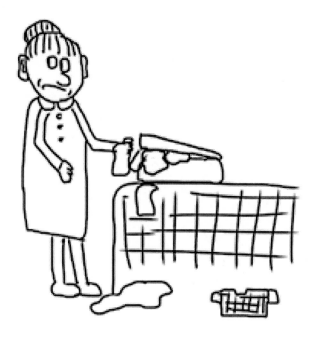

Turning I see a very young girl peeping in the door. She seems to be only a child. I stop momentarily as I glance her way. What on earth does she want? Scowling I decide the best alternative is to say nothing. The little wench will just go away. Oh my, where am I getting those awful words? Where do they come from?!?!? I don't say or think things like that.

I instinctively grab my head once again. Stop. Stop. Stop.

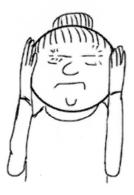

A voice interrupts my thoughts. The young girl is starting to say something.

"Irene it's breakfast time," the young girl says.

I turn away while continuing to ignore her. I don't need their breakfast. I just went to the supermarket a couple of days ago. I have a kitchen full of food items waiting, and nothing brews coffee like my old fashioned coffee kettle. I'll eat when I get home if my daughter hasn't cleaned me out of food. I go ahead and give a final heave and lift my suitcase. Turning to leave the room, I see that the young girl has now entered. Why won't she leave me alone? Doesn't she know this is a very important day? She continues to talk as she approaches me and I continue to scowl.

"Irene we have hot oat meal with brown sugar and melted butter—your breakfast favorite. I've already prepared your coffee the way you like it-2 creamers and 1 sugar. I'll walk to the dining room with you before it gets cold," she says as she reaches to take away my suitcase.

"Just the way I like it?" The words echo silently in my mind.

How does she know how I like my coffee? I don't like any coffee unless it is poured in a mug at my kitchen table within the solitude of my house! I feel the suitcase starting to slip out of my hands and quickly jerk it back.

"NO!!" I shout aloud.

Temporarily the young girl looks warily at me and then she begins again.

"Why don't you put your suitcase where you would like it to be and then you will know exactly where it is when you return from the dining room?"

"But I'm not going to the dining room with you," I say silently to myself.

Don't you know I am going home? My car is just right there. This is all a mistake. I turn away from the young child and point to the window where I see the morning light is starting to now reflect off my car's windshield. I continue to point. Surly she can see that is my car.

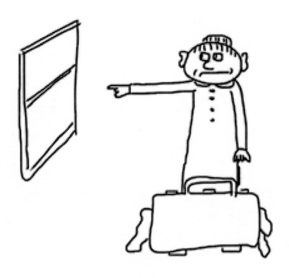

Yet, try as I might to relay the urgency of my departure, all I seem to mutter to her is, "Home-I want to go home."

"I know Irene. I know you want to go home. We all would like for you to be able to go home also. I know you have some pictures of your home in your drawer. Maybe we can look at them after breakfast together," the young girl says.

"NOT HUNGRY!" I yell as I get more and more frustrated that the young girl is so blind to the immediacy of my situation.

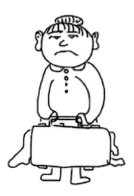

"Oh God," I silently plead. Why is this happening to me? I only want to be at home.

Tears start to run down my face and I feel my suitcase slipping out of my hand once again as I move my hands to wipe them away. To my dismay my suitcase flies open and my belongings are sprawled on the floor.

I want to scream, "Now look what you have done."

Yet those words seem to die on my tongue and I manage only to whimper, "No, no, no, no, no."

I grab my head and grip it tightly in a desperate gesture to control my mind. Closing my eyes, I begin to rock back and forth.

"No, no, no, no," I continue aloud.

Slowly I open my eyes. I stop rocking and glance downwards. All my precious and neatly stored things are strewn for all to see. What has my life become? Urging my arthritic knees to cooperate, I kneel slowly to start rectifying the mess when I suddenly spot my small silver case of lipstick. I reach to pick it up when I note that the young girl has also stooped to help. She too has seen the shiny cosmetic case and reaches for it.

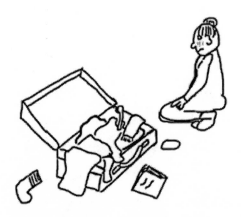

Holding it out to me she says, "Oh, look Irene it's your lipstick. You have been wondering where this was for several days. Now you can stick it back in your pocket where you keep it."

The young girl drops it into my hand and moments pass while I continue to only stare at the small object. My head starts to pound. I feel overwhelmingly tired. This is just too much for me. Can't anyone see this fiasco is killing me? I bow my head and tears again roll down my face. Exhaustion is overtaking me.

I look up to see the young girl waiting patiently. She places her hand on my shoulder in a gesture of comfort.

"Irene, why don't we get some breakfast and maybe you will feel better after you've eaten? Your daughter called this morning and said she would stop by and see you around 10 o'clock this morning. I can help get these things back in order while you have something to eat."

Suddenly the tears stop and my frustration turns again to anger with the absurdity of this entire situation. I want to yell at this young naïve child. I want to tell her that my daughter is the problem. This young girl is the problem. Everybody is the problem. They treat me like I don't know what I am doing

25

and have this superficial sense of sweetness about them-as if they think they are trying to help me.

Yet for some reason the words forsake me and I end up just shouting at the young girl, "No!!"

The young girl looks taken aback momentarily. She then stands and silently holds out her hand waiting for me to take it.

Well two can play at this game. I'll eat their breakfast and then quickly return to this room to pack and be gone before my daughter arrives.

A low groan escapes me as my arthritic knees allow me to cautiously stand again. I take the young girl's hand. I'll let her think she has won. Wordlessly, I accompany her out of the room and down a hallway.

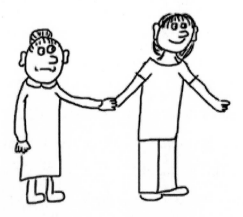

She escorts me to a seat at a round table where other unfamiliar women are already beginning to drink coffee and partake of their breakfast.

Once seated, I pick up a cup of coffee. I start to sip when one of the other ladies comments, "Good morning Irene. I hope you are well. We were beginning to worry about you. They have your favorite; oatmeal with brown sugar and butter."

Placing my coffee down I silently acknowledge this stranger by politely smiling. She thinks she knows me but I have never met her. She must have mistaken me for someone else. Oh well, better not to embarrass her and call it to her attention, and besides my daughter is probably paying her to keep an eye on me. In silence I pick up my spoon and start to delve into the creamy oatmeal. Steam rises from the bowl and the sugar has melted evenly on top. Then abruptly I stop. I wonder how much they are charging me for this meal. Brown sugar is quite expensive these days. I'm not sure I will have the money to pay these people for this meal until I get home and see what my daughter has done with my bank account. I place the unused spoon back beside the hot cereal bowl and return my napkin to the table to signify to these people that I don't want their meal. I steadily gaze ahead. Within my peripheral vision I see the young child approaching and hear her question me.

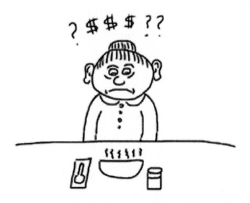

"Irene, aren't you hungry? You haven't touched your meal. Do you need some help? Here, let me stir it for you a little."

The young girl reaches for the spoon. If they see that I have partaken of their meal then they will charge me for it and I don't have the money. I grab the young girl's wrist before she can dirty the utensil and shout at her, "No!!"

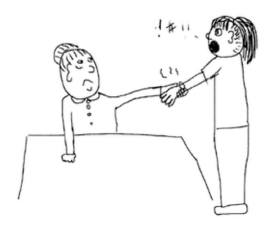

My grip tightens on her wrist and my anger again flares as my frustration mounts. None of this would be happening if they would just let me go home. I look up at the young girl to convey this to her. I don't want to hurt her. I start to explain but again all that comes out is, "Want home. Spoodles and tunes. Spoodles and tunes."

I see the young girl's wrist turning red underneath my grip. She calmly takes her other hand and pats me as if to reassure me. "Irene, it's okay if you're not hungry. We will save it for you and warm it. Can you let go and I will help you back to your room?"

My room? I look at her blankly and then release her wrist. I don't have a room here. What is she talking about?

I hear a young man approach and he quietly questions the young girl, "Do you want me to get Irene something to calm her down?"

My head is pounding by now. I am hungry but I fear eating. Why can I not figure this out? How did it come to all this? Why can I not figure this out? For goodness sake, I teach high school literature every day of my life. I have mastered Shakespeare, Hawthorne, and Conrad. Why can I not figure this out?

I hear the young girl tell the young gentleman, "No, the night shift said she didn't sleep well last night and was up packing most of the time. Let me see if she will take a nap and rest."

The young girl turns to me and holds out her hand. "Ready Irene?" she asks. "Let's walk back to your room. You seem really tired this morning."

I reach for her hand and stand. Rising fully to my feet, I panic when I realize that I have accidentally let some urine escape.

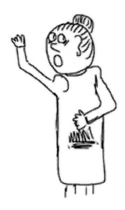

I feel my soiled undergarments and in shame look around to see if others are watching. If I walk with the young girl they will also see the 'tell-tell' signs of my accident. I drop her hand immediately as if it burned my skin and fall back into my chair.

"No!!" I shout at her. I steadily gaze ahead. If I ignore these people maybe they will just go away. I don't want to be here! How humiliating. I have these accidents at times, but when I am at home I can take care of them privately and no one is ever aware. I will sit here until I figure out what to do.

The young girl pats my shoulder once again. "Let me finish helping Mrs. Tomkins then and I will be back."

I watch as the young girl returns to a lady seated in a wheelchair at an adjacent table and begins to assist the elderly woman to eat. The woman is obviously an invalid and cannot lift her utensils.

This is a place for people like that, but I'm no invalid. I can walk and take care of myself. I can even drive. Drive? My mind clicks. My car-- I must get to my car and get out of here.

My thoughts are disrupted by a voice beside me. The stranger seated at my table is once again talking to me. "Irene, why don't you eat your toast if nothing else? Your daughter always comes in the morning and is worried when you haven't eaten."

"My daughter?" The words echo within my mind. I turn to this stranger seated beside me. My thoughts are refocused from my car to those two words-my daughter. So.... this lady is in on this after all. She probably reports everything to my filthy stealing daughter. Wonder how much she gets paid for the information? And to think, this stranger is probably getting paid out of MY money!!

Turning in my chair to squarely face her, I no longer pay heed to my soiled wet clothing. I rise to my full height of 5 feet 7 inches and look down upon the stranger. She continues to point to my untouched plate of food and encourages, "Just take a few bites."

"No!" I again scream while jerking my arm back and preparing to strike. I hit the lady hard with my fist. "My money. My money. My money."

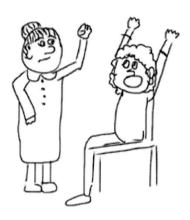

I hear people running towards me while saying, "Mrs. Carter. Mrs. Carter. Are you okay?"

I frantically look around. Who is Mrs. Carter?

Then others are running towards our table from a hall.

"Irene please stop," I hear someone command.

Looking down I see that the strange woman is developing a bruise on her check where only moments before my fist had slammed into her face. What could have possessed me? I am not a mean person. I sink down in the chair and tears flood my eyes.

"I want to go home," I manage to eke out in a desperate and weary voice.

"I don't want her in my house," I say while pointing to the strange woman beside me who is receiving only sympathy and compassion from these people. Don't they understand she is in on my daughter's scheme to take my money?

"Take her back to her room," I hear the gentleman who earlier was talking to the young girl say. I look around to find that he is directing the comment to me.

"No!!" I say.

Yet it is too late. Two strangers gather on either side of me and place an arm on either of my elbows and gently motion for me to stand with them. I stand in shame. My clothes are now further soiled and I must walk with them while everyone stares once again.

"Spoodles and tunes. Spoodles and tunes. Spoodles and tunes," I repeat aloud as I walk with them in total humiliation down the hallway. What has my life become?

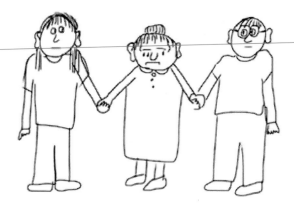

I arrive at a door which they open for me and enter a room I don't recognize. Walking in I find someone has left a suitcase on the bed. Someone must be moving in this room and they have obviously not finished unpacking.

"We'll be right back Irene. Stay here and let us check on Mrs. Carter," one of them directs.

Who is Mrs. Carter? I walk into the still and silent room. My urine soaked undergarments are beginning to cause much discomfort. I must change quickly and hide the undergarments so I will not get in trouble. I am not familiar with rules at this place, but if they think I soil my clothing I may get in trouble.

Walking to the drawers I rummage around. All of the undergarments look different than the ones I am accustomed

35

to wearing, but a pair will just have to work. Picking a plain cotton pair I note that it has my name in it. Why would someone have written my name in their undergarments?

I take the clean undergarment and enter the bathroom. I stop abruptly.

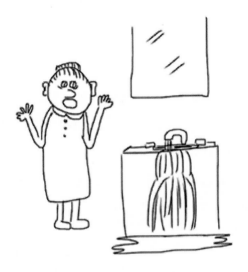

Where did all this water come from? Who would be so careless to leave water running? It has puddled in the floor. I gasp to myself. These people…these people….they will think I did this. They will tell my daughter and then I will never get to go home. I grab my head and rock.

"Think Irene. Think Irene," I again silently coax myself.

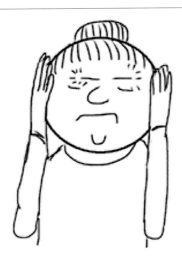

Wading through the water I make it to a paper towel dispenser and start rapidly pulling sheet after sheet from the dispenser. In huge stacks I cover the water. I turn the water off and look around. Piles of stacked wet paper towels are strewn everywhere, but it appears to be okay now. It is the best I can do. I will just pray no one will see it and tell my daughter. Exiting the bathroom I go into a corner of the room.

Removing my soiled clothing, I quickly change into dry clothing. I then take the soiled clothing and look through several drawers before finding a corner of one which I think will work. Wadding up my urine soiled clothing I push my dirty clothing items into the furthermost corner of the drawer. As I push the drawer closed I notice an awful odor permeates the drawer. I must get out of here. This place is not clean. This drawer reeks.

Closing the drawer tightly I feel assured no one will find the evidence of my accident.

Turning I notice a suitcase is on the bed. I don't want people to accuse me of stealing. This room is definitely meant for someone else. They must have just moved into it. They left their suitcase on the bed. I must find another room to gather my thoughts before the owner catches me.

I leave the room and walk three doors down the hall. None look familiar, but then again I have only been here for a few days. Opening the 4th door on the right I enter and find no one inside. I hesitantly look around.

There are pictures within the room, but I recognize none. Turning to leave I see a very used poetry book on a nightstand table.

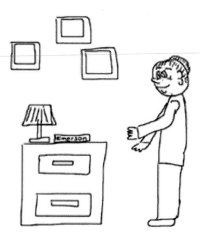

"Aw," I say to myself. It is my favorite book of poems. Memories flood my mind. Often are the days that I try to instill within my 11th grade students at Forest Oak High the appreciation of poetry. I read to them from this same book each day. How did it get here? I just had it yesterday in my home.

Picking up the book, I start to rummage through the pages. Just holding a poetry book brings comfort. A calm begins to overtake me as familiar poetic passages flood my mind.

"The greatest glory in living lies not in never falling, but in rising every time we fall." How many times did I quote that to my class?

My head is still heavy. I must not have slept well last night. Looking at the bed I decide to lie down for just five minutes. If I can just close my eyes for a few minutes then I can get my thoughts together and then I feel assured I will be able to make a plan to get out of here. Clutching my familiar book, I lie on the bed and hold it next to me. I am so tired.

Just five minutes. Just five minutes.

"Ah!!!!!" I startle awake to hear a piecing scream.

I sit up on the side of the bed and my dear copy of famous poetry falls to the floor.

"Get her out of my room." I hear another strange woman shouting and pointing at me. She is dressed in a red blouse and her face has turned the same shade of red as her blouse. She hatefully directs again, "Get her out of my room."

Reaching to rescue my fallen book, I once again grasp it to me tightly. I must have fallen asleep. My mind is circling and circling. I have to figure this out. I have to figure this out. I have to figure this out. Dear Lord, help me figure this out.

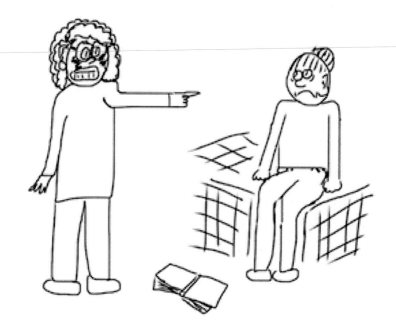

More strangers are entering the room and seem to be showing sympathy to this lady who is attired in red. They look at me in a reproachful manner and one speaks rather sharply.

"Irene. This is not your room. Come with me."

Another person lays their hand on the shoulder of the lady attired in red. "Calm down Mrs. Dickerson. Irene is confused. She didn't mean to disturb your room. We will help her out."

"I want my book back," demands the lady attired in red.

My mind continues to race. I must figure this out. I must figure this out. The conversation is going much too fast for me. Please Lord, help them to slow down for just a minute so I can gather my wits.

"I want my book now," the lady in red again insists.

Looking down at my cherished book of poems I pull it against me. A young girl approaches me again.

In a sweet and coaxing voice she says, "Irene, may I have Mrs. Dickerson's book back?"

"Not in never falling, but in rising....." My voice trails off as I fail to finish my cherished passage which I quote to my classroom students so often.

"Did you fall Ms. Irene?" The young girl stoops by the bed and looks up at me while I continue to sit on the side of the bed clutching my book.

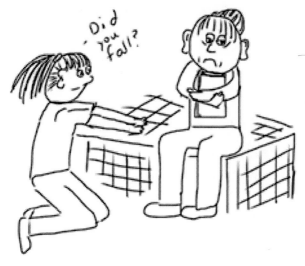

"Every time we fall," I finally manage to finish.

The young girl doesn't seem to understand. It is my book. I am able to quote from it. Doesn't she see? I am able to quote from it!! I know this book so well. It is truly mine. I would not lie.

Gently taking the book out of my grasps, the young girl turns to the inner cover. She points to a handwritten inscription and reads aloud to me, "To Mrs. Gladys Dickerson. May you always cherish these poems."

I look at the inscription and then back to the young lady's face turned up to me. This makes no sense. My book- my cherished passages- Is she saying it has someone else's name in it?

"Fall," is all I manage to say. Tears well up in my eyes. I am so tired.

"Fall, fall, fall, fall," I continue. I begin to rock back and forth while seated on the bed.

"Come on Ms. Irene. Let's go back to your room." The young girl stands and extends her hand to me.

My knees are exceedingly sore as I try to stand. I must get home and take my Tylenol. They have no idea how I hurt here. I have none of my medicine or things here to make me comfortable and I am sure there is a rule that I must pay for extra items such as medicine.

"Are you okay Ms. Irene? Are you hurting?" the young girl asks as she watches me gingerly take a step.

I just look at her in silence. What good does it do to answer? My gait steadies as I start to walk more and I manage to follow her wherever it is she is leading me.

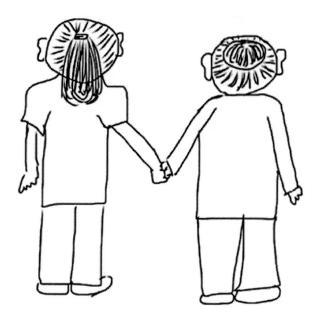

We arrive at a room where there is a suitcase on the bed. That is strange. I had a dream it seems recently about a suitcase and things spread all over the floor.

A lady with a mop and pail is coming out of the bathroom as we enter the room. She comments to the young girl, "Melody, I want you to know water and paper towels were all over the bathroom floor again. Ms. Irene leaves the water running in her bathroom every morning and then tries to clean it herself."

Why is this person with a mop looking at me as if I am to blame for her task of cleaning the bathroom? I glare back at her. That is the job of school custodians. I don't understand why she is acting like I have done something wrong. Why, I don't even know whose classroom this is. I always leave mine in a very orderly condition at the end of the school day. It's probably Mr. Gillman's chemistry class. His lab is always disorganized. Well, I am not going to get fired for his mistake. I'll just let the school custodian know it's Gillman's mess.

Turning to face the lady with the mop I scowl at her and yell, "Mess Gillmans."

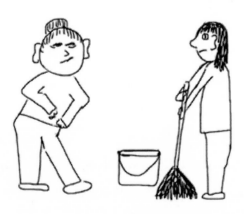

I see the young girl coming to intervene. She is probably going to take the custodian's side. She places her hand gently on my shoulder and in a quiet voice says, "It's okay Irene. I don't know Miss Gillmans. I'm sure she is nice. This is Mrs. Dennings and she wanted to be nice also. She just finished cleaning the bathroom."

"Thank you Mrs. Dennings," the young girl says while turning to the school custodian. She then motions for the custodian to leave.

The young girl gently moves her hand from my shoulder to my hand and prompts with a gentle tug to walk closer to a bed in the room.

Why is there a bed in Gillman's chemistry lab, and one with a suitcase? Articles of clothing are spilling over from the poorly packed suitcase. Someone must have been in a hurry. I watch as the young girl places the suitcase in a closet and pulls down the bed covers. This is too much for me. I don't understand. I am so tired. Will I get in trouble if I lie down? Will the principal catch me and I lose my job?

I hear another person entering behind me. It's a young gentleman. I hear him say, "I went ahead and got something for Irene."

Then he approaches me with a container. The cup must belong in Mr. Gillman's lab, and this man is returning it. I try to tell him I don't teach chemistry. This isn't even my classroom. He can take that concoction away from me, but this time I am so tired and I only manage to shake my head back and forth. Words entirely fail me.

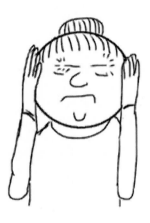

Now the gentleman is spooning something out of the cup and holding it up to my mouth while saying something. I am so tired. I don't even hear his voice-it is completely blocked. I just shake my head back and forth...back and forth...back and forth. I close my eyes. Back and forth and back and forth my head goes. I shut my lips tighter and tighter. I swing my head back and forth faster and faster. Stop. Stop. Stop. Stop. Stop. My mind is circling and circling.

Then I hear the young girl's voice again. For some reason her words come through to my weary mind. Her voice has a familiarity about it.

"Come on Ms. Irene. You didn't eat your breakfast and Luke has brought you a little applesauce so you won't be hungry. You always rest better if you are not hungry. Then you will be able to take a nap and feel all better. You must be so tired."

My head stops and I open my eyes. This young girl seems sweet. She seems so much nicer than the rest. I feel she is the only one wanting to help me. I am tired…so tired. For a few seconds I hesitate as I try to figure out what I should do before I finally decide to open my mouth. I swallow the concoction being lifted to my mouth by this strange man. For some reason it is very bitter and grainy.

I look back at the young girl. Have I done what she wants? Maybe if I do what she asks then she will help me. Maybe she is the one I can trust. For some reason her face seems like an honest one. At times I almost feel like I know her. She must be in my English class.

I start to climb into the bed as the young girl walks to a dresser within the room and opens a drawer. Reaching inside she removes a heavily worn red book. As she approaches my bed she hands the well loved book to me and says, "Here Ms. Irene. Here is your book."

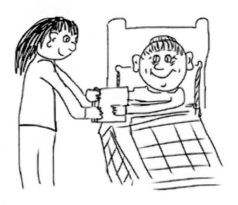

I reach for the book entitled, "Famous Poems Of Famous Poets." I slip it under my pillow where no one can steal it and then I close my heavy eyes. I am so tired..so tired.

Wild dreams overtake my mind as I doze in a fitful sleep. I find myself in my familiar 11th grade English high school classroom. There are many students and I do not feel prepared to teach as I usually do. The students seem to know more than I do. What if the principal finds that my mind is slipping? Will I lose my job? In my dream I gasp as I see my daughter seated in the front row. What is she doing in my classroom? She is raising her hand and I decide to ignore her. I direct the class to turn to page 112 in their American Literature book.

My daughter again raises her hand. Without gaining permission to speak she questions aloud, "Mother, don't you think this is getting a little too much for you?"

In my dream I look at her in dismay. My own daughter is turning against me.

The rest of the class begins to snicker and I hear them begin to whisper, "Too much. Too much. Too much."

I break out in a sweat. What am I going to do? People will find out I am having a little trouble remembering.

Then I feel something soothing on my forehead. It is a hand and it is stroking my hair back. This is not part of my dream. Someone is here with me, but my eyes are so heavy and I can't see who it is.

I hear what seems a gentle and familiar voice in the distance saying, "It's okay Mom. I'm here. Just try to rest."

I partially open my eyes and see my sister sitting by my bed. She is so young again. I hear her say, "It's going to be okay."

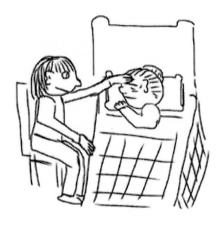

My head feels heavy like I have been drugged, but if my sister is here everything will be okay. Before I start to slip back to sleep I hear another person's voice. The voice seems to be speaking to my sister Janice. The voice is calling Janice by the wrong name, but I am too tired to correct the mistake.

I hear the voice say, "Janette, the first shift nurse gave your mom some Ativan in some applesauce to help her rest for a while. She was up packing a suitcase all night and the staff couldn't redirect her or calm her. She flooded the bathroom this morning, but thankfully didn't fall in the water. Then she appeared agitated all morning and hit another resident who didn't even provoke her while in the dining room. Later we found her asleep in Mrs. Dickerson's room. She mostly talked about falling, but we haven't been able to determine if she fell or not. She has no bruises. She is just a little more agitated today it seems. Your mom seems to respond best to Melody. Melody has taken care of her for the past year, and finally Melody was able to coax her into resting. She has been sleeping since around 9:45 this morning but in a restless way."

I feel the comforting hand of my sister still stroking my forehead as I once again hear the familiar voice answering. "I'm sorry Mom was so agitated. Please tell your staff to call me anytime during the night. I will stay for a while. She seems to be calming down now. Then I will come back tonight and check on her."

"Sounds good," the other unfamiliar voice replies. "Oh, one more thing-I cleaned out her 4th drawer and bagged her soiled clothing for you to launder at home. It's in the bathroom now. She keeps hiding her soiled clothing in that particular drawer and we will try to get the odor out."

"Thanks. I understand. I'll grab the laundry on the way out."

I once again partially open my eyes and see my sister Janice still beside me. Her hand remains comforting as she continues to stroke my head. Knowing she is there I decide it is safe to just close my eyes again. I will figure it all out later. It is just too much for me and I am so tired. I close my eyes and finally drift off to a restful sleep.

When I awaken it appears to be late afternoon. I find myself in a strange room. Something has left an indention on my head where I slept. Reaching my hand behind the pillow, I find I have slept on a book. Now why is a book under my pillow? I place it on the bedside and slowly sit up. My body aches. My arthritis is winning a battle. If I don't get home soon and back to my daily walking exercises in my yard and my routine Tylenol, I won't be able to move.

I coax my feet to the window and look out. I spy a nice shiny Buick parked three spaces from my window. My car!! It's my car. I must get home. I fumble through my pockets. Where are my keys? I find only a cosmetic case and a piece of paper with a written notation in my pocket. I struggle to read the extremely worn and crumpled paper. The piece of paper looks as if it was written years ago. Why do I have it in my pocket? Puzzling for a moment, I drop it on the floor and delve deeper into my pockets but disappointedly I find no keys.

I think I must have left them in the car. I glance out the window again. Yes, the car is still there. I will go now and find out. I wonder if I should pack anything but hurriedly ruffling through my drawers I find that none of my things are here anyway.

I just have to get out of here. Heading to the door I stop to again reflect on the worn piece of paper which had been in my pocket and which is now on the floor. I slowly stoop and pick it up. I don't understand what it is or why I had it, but wonder if it is important? It might have some information about my bank accounts. I stuff it back in my pocket and decide I'll look at it again when I get home. I am sure I will be able to make sense of it there when I can think clearly. Besides I don't want these people finding out too much about me.

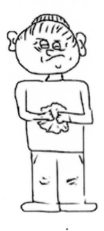

I walk to the door and glance down the hallway. No one is around as I head to the end of the hallway. I start to push on a door that looks like it might lead to the parking lot. But before my hand touches the horizontal exit bar, I abruptly stop. For some reason I feel like I have done this before and I have an uneasy feeling there is something I must do before I touch the bar.

"Think Irene. Think Irene," I silently coax myself.

Someone will be coming down the hall soon. I have to figure this out. Habitually I raise my arms as I start to grab my head in a desperate gesture to control my thoughts. As my arm passes by my line of vision I spy a gray bracelet on my left wrist.

I stop. I look at the bracelet. There is an uneasy feeling about this bracelet and although I don't know why I would think this I begin to wonder if this bracelet has something to do with this door.

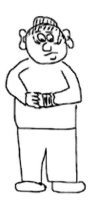

I look from the bracelet to the door and then from the door to the bracelet. I tug at the bracelet in an effort to remove it from my wrist.

"Damn it!" I cry aloud. Where did that word come from? I don't say words like that. I look around to see if anyone heard. The hall is still empty.

I again look at the door. How many times in my life have I walked through a door? This one door is the only thing keeping me from my car and yet for some reason I feel there is something different about this door, but what is it?

Then for a fraction of a second I feel clarity in knowing the bracelet on my wrist must not be near the door if it is to open. I am unsure why I know this, but I just do. If the bracelet is near the door then there will be a click and the bar will lock down. Is this true? Am I right? Please Lord let me be right.

Using my height and my arm span to an advantage I turn sideways to the door. I lift my left arm so that the bracelet clad wrist is in the farthermost position from the door. I then reach with my uplifted right arm and press on the door.

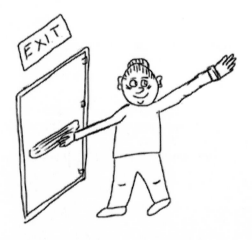

I do not hear a clicking lock. I push. The door opens. Joy fills my soul. It worked. The door is open. The door is open. I am almost to my car. Now that the door is open I pay no heed to being wary of the bracelet and rush to get through. My arm swings down to my side again. As I walk by the door frame a deafening noise rings everywhere around me.

"Weeeeooh..weeeeooh....Weeeeooh." An alarm is ringing. I cover my ears completely. What have I done?

"Please Lord," I silently plead. I am so close. I am so close. My car should be right here. This nightmare is almost over.

Once outside I realize it is becoming rather late in the afternoon. I start to panic. I will just walk. I am sure my car is around this corner. I feel assured I will spot it in a minute. Suddenly I hear voices shouting behind me in the distance.

"Stop Irene. Come back," I hear one of them command.

I find my arthritic knees are newly spurred on by fear that these shouting people are going to stop me for some reason. With more haste than ever before, I continue walking. The footsteps and voices are gaining on me.

Where is my car? I know it is here. I frantically look back and forth. I have to make a decision soon which way to go. A ball of fear knots up in my stomach. I am so close. I have to figure this out. Which direction is my car? My freedom is so close!

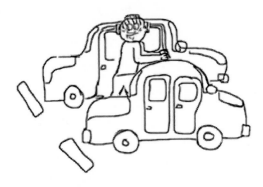

I hear another voice with a sense of urgency shout, "Irene, wait! There are cars entering the driveway."

Not knowing what to do I head for a wooded area and walk away from the paved area. There are too many cars for me to find mine. I can't think with these people shouting at me. My knees are starting to hurt now and my walking is more shuffled. If I can get into the woods then I will find a private place to think and figure this out. I just need to be quiet for a few moments and it will come to me….the location of my car. I will hide from the people chasing me.

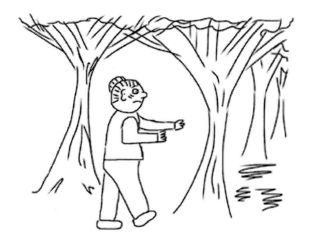

I look over my shoulder once again as I enter the wooded area to make sure they are not following me. Turning to face forward I realize too late I have misjudged the ground. There is a hill at the edge of the woods and I feel a tear in my leg as I fall. I land haphazardly and stunned at the bottom.

Strangers are rushing toward me. Looking down I see bright blood seeping from underneath my pants leg. In my bathroom medicine cabinet at home I have lots of things. I will ask these people coming toward me to help me find my car and explain I have some band-aides at home. Surly they will see that it is very important I get home now. I need to stop the bleeding.

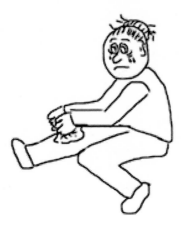

"Ms. Irene. Are you okay?" I hear someone ask as they get closer to me.

I look up at her. This sweet girl seems familiar. She falls to her knees beside me and again I see what appears to be concern in her eyes.

I start to explain to her that I am fine and that my band-aides are at home, but somehow the only words I form are "home, bathroom."

A strange gentleman arrives and begins to pull up my pants leg. I don't know this man. I take my fist and swipe at him as he is bending over me. I don't want some strange man looking at my legs.

"No! No! NO!" I say as I again flail at him.

He backs away and the young girl bends toward me once again.

"Irene, Jack needs to look at your leg and stop the bleeding. Please Ms. Irene, will you let him help you?"

Help me? Help me!? If anyone wanted to help me they would just let me go. That is all I need.

I push the young girl away a little more gently. She seems nicer than the rest of these strangers and I attempt to stand. Although difficult I manage to get half way to a standing position when suddenly everything turns black and my last thought is of falling once more and someone catching me.

I awake in a strange bed. Where am I? I turn over but feel a sharp pain in my leg. In the background I hear the soft melody of my favorite classical musical piece, "Claire de Lune." I look around to find a vinyl record spinning around on my record player. The soothing melody brings back good memories.

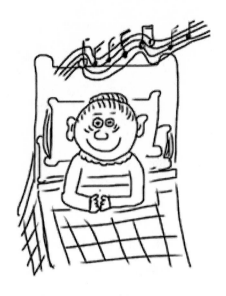

"Tunes," I say aloud.

"Yes Mom," I hear a voice say.

Turning to the right I see my sister again. She's here!!

"Oh Janice I am so tired and so glad you are here," I think silently to myself.

Janice approaches and lays a hand on my shoulder.

Tenderly she looks down at me and says, "I got the needle replacement for your stereo the other day. Nothing like the vinyl sound as you always said. Don't your classical tunes sound nice, Mom?"

"Tunes," I say again and smile back at her.

"Here Mom, the doctor says it's okay if you prop up in bed for a few minutes."

My sister starts to help me sit up slightly in bed and fluff the pillows behind me.

"I've got another surprise," my sister continues. "I talked to Melody and she said you didn't sleep well last night. I think my surprise might help you rest a little better tonight. I'm going to stay with you and I brought a guest which Melody says is okay for one night."

The classical music is starting to help me focus. I see my sister turn and call out towards a hidden alcove in the room.

"Come on old girl. Here Spoodles," my sister calls.

"Spoodles?" I silently repeat in my mind.

Out from the dark recess of the room I spy a miniature black ball of fur emerge. I smile to myself as I recognize my old friend and loyal companion coming closer.

I hold out my arms and cry out, "Spoodles, Spoodles, Spoodles!"

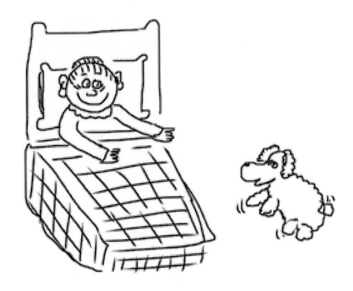

But my dear friend is not jumping up like she always does.

I see my sister bend and pick her up before then placing her on my bed beside me.

"She's getting like the rest of us Mom," my sister laughs and adds, "a little old. In December Spoodles will be 14 years old. I still laugh when I think about Madison that Christmas day telling you, 'I like your Spoodles Grammy.' Madison will be 19 years old this year and Spoodles here will soon turn 14."

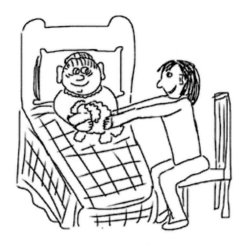

I feel Spoodles curling up beside me as she does every day. I pat her head and memories again flood my mind. Spoodles has been my dearest companion. She is the only one in whom I confide. Sometimes I whisper and tell her that I am worried I am getting a little forgetful. I know my secret will be safe with her.

The album is continuing to fill the room with the soft sound of classical music. I don't recognize this room, but for the moment it doesn't matter because Spoodles and my sister are by my side.

"Just lean back and rest Mom," my sister says quietly.

She is pulling up a chair beside me.

"I will be here all night. It's going to be okay."

My sister places her hand on my shoulder as if in a gesture of reassurance.

With my hand still resting on Spoodles I look up to see my sister smile at me and she says, "I love you, Mom."

Then for the briefest of all moments....for a fraction of a second..... my thoughts are not confused and I experience momentary recognition as I feel my daughter's love. This isn't my sister. This is Janette, my beloved daughter.

"I love you too Janette," I clearly say and smile back.

She reaches for my hand and squeezes it tightly. I am tired. Her touch feels good.

I will close my eyes for just a few minutes and rest. I snuggle back into my propped pillows and my last thoughts before going to sleep are about how nice it is to see my sister and Spoodles, but tomorrow I must get out of here. Tomorrow I must make a plan.

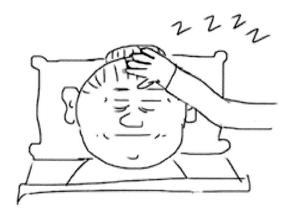

The End

Wouldn't it be wonderful if one simple story could generate a large amount of research money for Alzheimer's disease and other dementia disorders? The possibility this will occur lies solely in the hands of our readers and their motivation to make a difference. They truly may hold the key in their hands. Undoubtedly there are amateur imperfections in this book, but we are hoping readers will look pass them and find Irene's story worthy to be shared. If you found meaning in the story and encourage others to also purchase the book, we would like to say, "Thank You!!!" Thank you for helping those individuals who can no longer ask for help, but who desperately need someone to care.

Jennifer Orsak and Amy Hurley

CPSIA information can be obtained
at www.ICGtesting.com
Printed in the USA
FFOW04n1607290716
26365FF